AMERICAN PUBLIC UNIVERSITY SYSTEM

AN EXPLORATION OF THE IMPLEMENTATION

AND ISSUES OF MANDATORY SEASONAL

INFLUENZA VACCINATION POLICY UNDER THE

SYSTEMS THEORY

A DISSERTATION SUBMITTED TO

THE FACULTY OF THE DIVISION OF THE SOCIAL

SCIENCES

IN CANDIDACY FOR THE DEGREE OF

MASTERS IN PUBLIC ADMINISTRATION

DEPARTMENT OF SECURITY AND GLOBAL

STUDIES

BY

MARY CONSTANTINE WACK

MARCH 2011

The author hereby grants the American Public University System the right to display these contents for educational purposes.

The author assumes total responsibility for meeting the requirements set by United States Copyright Law for the inclusion of any materials that are not the author's creation or in the public domain.

DEDICATION

I dedicate my dissertation to all the health care workers who devote their time, caring, and compassion to the public's health. We could not survive without you.

ACKNOWLEDGEMENTS

I would like to thank the faculty and staff of American

Public University System and my family for their continued

support, knowledge, and devotion to education.

ABSTRACT OF THE RESEARCH PAPER

AN EXPLORATION OF THE IMPLEMENTATION

AND ISSUES OF MANDATORY SEASONAL

INFLUENZA VACCINATION POLICY UNDER THE

SYSTEMS THEORY

by

Mary Constantine Wack

American Public University System, March 25, 2011

Charles Town, West Virginia

Professor Herbert Brown, Thesis Professor

This study explores the implementation of
mandatory seasonal influenza vaccination policy for health
care workers at BJC Healthcare, a large Midwestern health
care organization of approximately 26,000 employees. The
purpose of this study is to gain insight into the effectiveness
and issues of mandatory seasonal influenza vaccination of
health care workers. A single-case study approach is
utilized, along with the systems theory as a theoretical

framework. By examining the implementation of mandatory seasonal influenza vaccination policy at BJC Healthcare, this study is able to categorize three potential areas of conflict under the systems theory: technology, the labor force, and the task environment. Discussion of these three sources of uncertainty and conflict allows for greater understanding of the issues of implementing mandatory seasonal influenza vaccination policy that need to be resolved in order to promote health care institution effectiveness, function, and successful implementation of mandatory seasonal influenza vaccination policy.

TABLE OF CONTENTS

Chapter

        Purpose and Signficance of the Study

        Research Questions

        Definition of Terms

        Nature of the Study or

        Theoretical/Conceptual Framework

        Introduction

        Research Design and Instrumentation

LIST OF TABLES

Table   Page

LIST OF FIGURES

CHAPTER 1

INTRODUCTION TO THE PROBLEM

Influenza is a highly contagious respiratory illness caused by influenza viruses. People can transmit the virus to each other up to 6 feet away through droplets in the air as they talk, sneeze, or cough.[1] In addition, influenza may be spread by touching a surface that has influenza virus on it, then touching his or her own mouth or nose. Once infected, a person can develop mild to severe symptoms, and an estimated average of 36,000 people die annually from influenza. Each year influenza epidemics cause 610,660 life-years lost, 3.1 million days of hospitalization, and 31.4 million outpatient visits.[2]

---

[1] "Seasonal Influenza (Flu)," *Centers for Disease Control and Prevention*, last modified September 15, 2010, http:/www.cdc.gov/flu.

[2] Michele L. Pearson, Carolyn B. Bridges, and Scott A. Harper, "Influenza Vaccination of Health-Care Personnel: Recommendations of the Healthcare Infection Control Practices Advisory Committee (HICPAC) and the Advisory Committee on Immunization Practices (ACIP)," *Morbidity and Mortality Weekly Report*, 55, no. 2 (2006): 1-16, http://www.cdc.gov/mmwr/preview/mmwrhtml/rr5502a1.htm.

Due to the high occurrence of influenza within health care institutions, including public agencies that provide health care, health care workers are at increased risk of acquiring and transmitting influenza to other staff, patients, and families. The best way to prevent the spread of influenza is the influenza vaccine, and Healthy People 2010 specifically targeted health care personnel as a special subset of the population that should receive the influenza vaccine. The new proposed goal for Healthy People 2020 is 90 percent coverage for health care worker influenza vaccination, which, as indicated by previous research, would lower the incidence of nosocomial influenza cases and staff abseentism.[3]

However, health care worker influenza vaccinations rates remain around 40 percent across the nation.[4] Although the two types of influenza vaccines, the

---

[3,4] "HHS Action Plan to Prevent Healthcare-Associated Infections: Influenza Vaccination of Healthcare Personnel," *U.S. Department of Health & Human Services*, last modified May 2010, http://www.hhs.gov/ash/initiatives/hai/tier2_flu.html.

inactivated vaccine, or the flu shot, and the attenuated vaccine, or nasal spray, are stringently regulated and deemed safe by the Food and Drug Administration (FDA), minor side effects such as soreness and swelling at the injection site and personal fears about the influenza vaccine have swayed many health care worker from receiving the influenza vaccine. Due to low influenza vaccination coverage of health care workers, some health care institutions have implemented mandatory seasonal influenza vaccination for health care workers. Under these mandatory seasonal influenza vaccination policies, any health care worker employed by the health care institution must receive the influenza vaccine by a certain date as a condition of employment. Noncompliance at the health care institutions with mandatory seasonal influenza vaccination policies results in termination of employment.

In 2005 Virginia Mason Medical Center became the first health care institution to implement mandatory seasonal influenza vaccination for health care workers.[5]

More than 25 other health care institutions have since

implemented similar policies, including Barnes-Jewish

Corporation (BJC) Healthcare, a system of 11 acute care

and 3 extended care facilities in the Midwest region. This

case study will review the implementation and

effectiveness of mandatory seasonal influenza vaccination

policy at BJC Healthcare, and this case study will also

explore the issues of mandatory seasonal influenza

vaccination as illustrated by BJC Healthcare and that may

occur in the future at BJC Healthcare and other public or

private health care institutions that implement mandatory

seasonal influenza vaccination for health care workers.

[5] Thomas R. Talbot and William Schaffner, "On Being the First: Virginia Mason Medical Center and Mandatory Influenza vaccination of Healthcare workers," *Infection Control Hospital Epidemiology*, 31, no. 9 (2010): 889-892, doi: 10.1086/656211.

CHAPTER 2

INTRODUCTION TO THE STUDY

Purpose and Significance of the Study

The importance of influenza vaccination among health care workers cannot be overestimated. Prevention of influenza among health care workers through vaccination can stop the spread of influenza to patients, families, and other staff, which in turn averts potential hospitalization, life-years lost, and death. This case study examines the implementation of mandatory seasonal influenza vaccinations of health care workers at BJC Healthcare, which implemented mandatory seasonal vaccinations for health care workers to increase vaccination coverage and consequently reduce employee illness, abseentism, and morbidity and mortality due to influenza. More specifically, this case study explores the effectiveness of mandatory seasonal influenza vaccination for health care workers at BJC Healthcare and sets out to gain insight into the issues or conflicts that arise or may arise at health care institutions that implement mandatory seasonal influenza vaccination policies.

The issues that this case study identifies as a direct or indirect consequence of the implementation of mandatory seasonal influenza vaccination for health care workers will be beneficial to health care organizations that embark on future implementation of mandatory seasonal influenza vaccination policies at their institutions. Knowing what possible complications to expect may help guide institutions in preparing better policies or preparing implementation guidelines to cope with the issues that may arise. These preparations will enhance the effectiveness of influenza vaccination as well as improve the function of the health care institutions in the future.

Research Questions

The following questions were researched in this study:

1. Does mandatory seasonal influenza vaccination of health care workers increase influenza vaccination coverage among health care workers?

2. What issues or conflicts occur during or after implementation of mandatory seasonal influenza vaccination of health care workers?

Definition of Terms

Mandatory seasonal influenza vaccination. An institution's requirement for its health care workers to receive seasonal influenza vaccination as a condition of employment.

Health care worker. All paid and unpaid people working in a health care setting who have possible exposure to infectious materials and are directly or indirectly involved in patient care.[6]

---

[6] "HHS Action Plan to Prevent Healthcare-Associated Infections: Influenza Vaccination of Healthcare Personnel," *U.S.*

Nature of the Study or Theoretical/Conceptual Framework

The theoretical framework for this case study centers on the theory that open systems, such as those found in health care, operate with interacting components toward a common purpose. Thus, under the systems theory, organizations take inputs from the environment, change them, and release them into the environment. The organization becomes a part of the environment in which it operates, and the two form a contingent cycle in which the organizations are dependent on the environment and the environment is dependent on organizations.[7] Moreover, the organization works with specialized, interdependent subsystems that are connected through such processes as management, communication, and feedback. Environmental forces and the organization and

---

Department of Health & Human Services, last modified May 2010, http://www.hhs.gov/ash/initiatives/hai/tier2_flu.html.

[7] Daniel Katz and Robert L. Kahn, "Organizations and the Systems Concept," in *Classics of Public Administration*, 6h ed. ed. Jay M. Shafritz and Albert Hyde (Boston, MA: Thomson Wadsworth, 2007), 189-198.

management controlling them, then, alter outputs and the reciprocating environment.

Furthermore, under the open systems theory, organizations must gain support from the environment to set goals. The role of administration in this theoretical construct is to direct decision processes and make choices to achieve these goals, which are complicated by the amount of agreement or disagreement among decision makers in their attitudes toward the causation of alternative actions and potential results.[8] Further conflict can arise due to three sources of uncertainty: the labor force, technology, or the task environment, which refers to characteristics of the environment that influence management decisions in regards to goal setting and goal realization. To accomplish optimal organizational effectiveness, organizations may use legal compliance, instrumental satisfaction or rewards, self

---

[8] James Thompson, *Organizations in Action: Social Science Bases of Administration Theory* (New York, NY: McGraw-Hill, 1962), quoted in John Miner, *Organizational behavior 2: Essential theories of process and structure* (Armonk, NY: M. E. Sharpe, Inc, 2006). PDF e-book.

expression, and internalization, as well as addressing the three sources of uncertainty and conflict that decrease organizational function.

Under the systems theory, health care organizations are open systems that are influenced by, and in turn influence, the environment. Both private and public health care organizations operate through management, communication, and feedback, and the implementation of mandatory seasonal influenza vaccination of health care workers follows this cycle. However, as the open systems theory demonstrates, organizations will encounter uncertainty and conflict as they implement the mandatory seasonal influenza vaccination policy due to three sources, which will be explore in this case study.

CHAPTER 3

RESEARCH DESIGN AND METHODS

Introduction

The purpose of this case study is to gain insight into the use, implementation, and issues of mandatory seasonal influenza vaccination for health care workers at health care institutions. As evidenced by the overview of influenza and vaccination, mandatory seasonal influenza vaccination policies for health care workers are becoming more common. In 2008 BJC Healthcare joined the growing number of health care institutions mandating seasonal influenza vaccination for health care workers. This research review is designed to explore the organization's history, implementation of mandatory seasonal influenza vaccination policy, and issues of mandatory seasonal influenza vaccination for health care workers to answer the two research questions of this case study under the systems theory as a theoretical framework.

Research Design and Instrumentation

This study is a case study utilizing information

gathered by BJC Healthcare in an effort to examine the

organization's implementation of mandatory seasonal

influenza vaccination for health care workers and explore

consequent issues of organization's implementation of such

policies. The data examines includes quantitative and

qualitative information. A case study formation is used

because case studies allow researchers to perform a detailed

exploration of a process, event, program, or one or more

individuals.[9] The natural setting of a case study encourages

researchers to experience the issue or problem being

explored, and an inductive data analytical process helps

researchers to create patterns, categories, and themes by

arranging the data into progressively more abstract

divisions of information to form a larger picture of the issue

under study. Furthermore, in the case study for this report,

---

[9] John W. Creswell, *Research Design: Qualitative, Quantitative, and Mixed Methods Approaches*, 3d ed. (Los Angeles, CA: SAGE Publications, Inc., 2009).

the single-case study is suitable for an exploration of the issue. Lessons learned through the case study are considered relevant and informative about the experiences of implementing mandatory seasonal influenza vaccination for health care workers.

Data Collection Procedures

This case study utilizes data collected from a BJC Healthcare study performed after the first year of mandatory seasonal influenza vaccination for health care workers at the organization. The data from the BJC Healthcare study was tabulated and presented in a table using descriptive statistics. An additional chart showing seasonal influenza vaccination rates among health care personnel at BJC Healthcare and the National Health Interview Survey rates over a course of 12 years was presented to compare vaccination rates pre- and post-policy. This case study also looks at thematic issues that emerged from the BJC Healthcare study during and after implementation of mandatory seasonal influenza

vaccination for the organization's health care workers.

CHAPTER 4

DATA COLLECTION AND ANALYSIS

Introduction

The purpose of this case study is to gain insight into the implementation and issues of mandatory seasonal influenza vaccination for health care workers. The selection of the case study represents one of the largest health care organizations in the U.S. to institute mandatory seasonal influenza vaccination for health care workers. The success of mandatory seasonal influenza vaccination at the health care organization of this study could influence the future of influenza vaccination at other private and public health care institutions. However, the issues that emerge during and after policy implementation as demonstrated by this case study could carry over into future implementation of mandatory seasonal influenza vaccination to either positively or negatively impact influenza rates at BJC Healthcare and similar institutions, private or public.

Organization History and Setting

BJC Healthcare is a large health care organization situated in Missouri and Illinois. The organization consists of approximately 26,000 employees throughout its 11 acute care hospitals, 3 extended care facilities, day care centers, home care, behavioral health services, and occupational medicine centers.[10] Prior to 2008, influenza rates of health care workers remained well below the targeted BJC rate of 80 percent. Therefore, in 2008 BJC Healthcare implemented a mandatory seasonal influenza vaccination policy for all health care employees.

As a patient safety initiative, the mandatory seasonal influenza vaccination focuses on all employees who are directly or indirectly involved in patient care,

---

[10] Hilary M. Babcock and others, eds, "Mandatory Influenza Vaccination of Health Care Workers: Translating Policy to Practice," *Clinical Infectious Diseases*, 50, no. 4 (2010): 459-464, doi: 10.1086/650752.

including clinical and nonclinical staff, hospital-employed physicians, volunteers, and contracted clinical workers. However, non-employees of BJC Healthcare are not covered by the policy and therefore are not mandated to receive seasonal influenza vaccination. This category includes attending physicians who are not employed by BJC Healthcare but are instead employed by Washington University School of Medicine, the physician group associated with BJC Healthcare, or are in private practice. Other exemptions to the mandatory seasonal influenza vaccination policy are granted on medical or religious exemptions.

In order to receive a religious exemption, employees must present a letter stating their religious conviction opposing vaccination to the Human Resources departments of BJC Healthcare. Similarly, employees requesting medical exemptions must have a letter from a physician stating a medical contraindication to the influenza vaccination, such as hypersensitivity to eggs, a history of Guillan-Barré syndrome, autoimmune or neurological condition concerns, or a previous hypersensitivity to the influenza vaccine. Letters from a physician recommending non-vaccination on the basis of pregnancy are also accepted. Once presented to Human Resources, occupational health nurses review the requests individually, and the employee requesting exemption receives a reply of exemption or denial within 5 days.

Policy Communication, Implementation, and Tracking

BJC Healthcare's mandatory seasonal influenza vaccination policy is communicated through several venues. These methods include through managerial communication and provision of education materials and fact sheets; letters in the mail; an internal Intranet site; the organization's in-house newspaper; and public meetings throughout the implementation phase of influenza vaccination with occupation health nurses, infectious disease physicians, and infection prevention specialists in attendance.

The inactivated and the live attenuated influenza vaccine are provided free to employees at multiple locations within BJC Healthcare. The implementation date starts in October and goes through December. Vaccine distribution is tracked at each facility of BJC Healthcare in real time through consent forms, badge scanners, and a database in which managers can enter in vaccinated employees. The database is then downloaded into the BJC occupational health database, and the occupation health departments provided weekly feedback to managers to encourage compliance with the policy. Employees not vaccinated by the end of the vaccination period are suspended with pay. If the suspended employee does not receive influenza vaccination by January of the following year, the employee is terminated.

Results

Quantitative Results

During the 2008 influenza vaccination season at BJC Healthcare, 25,980 health care workers were required to receive seasonal influenza vaccination. 25, 561 employees received the influenza vaccine, while 411 employees were exempted from influenza vaccination.[11] 99.96 percent of employees, then, were compliant with the mandatory seasonal influenza vaccination policy. The 0.03 percent of employees, or 8 employees, noncompliant with the influenza vaccination policy were terminated.

372 employees requested medical exemption, but only 321 medical exemptions were granted by occupational health on the basis of allergy to eggs; prior hypersensitivity to the influenza vaccine; history of Guillan-Barré syndrome; pregnancy; neurologic condition; autoimmune

---

[11] Hilary M. Babcock and others, eds, "Mandatory Influenza Vaccination of Health Care Workers: Translating Policy to Practice," *Clinical Infectious Diseases*, 50, no. 4 (2010): 459-464, doi: 10.1086/650752.

disease trigger; veganism; multiple food sensitivities; or

risk of rejection of transplanted organ.

Vaccination status	No. (%) of employees
Vaccinated	25,561 (98.4)
Religious exemption granted	90 (0.35)
Medical exemption granted	321 (1.24)
Egg allergy	107
Prior reaction and/or allergy to other component	83
History of Guillan-Barré syndrome	15
Other	116
Policy compliant (vaccinated or exempt)	25,972 (99.96)
Noncompliant (neither vaccinated or exempt)	8 (0.03)
Total employees	25,980

Table 1. Clinical Infectious Diseases, 2010.

The influenza vaccination rate at BJC Healthcare in

2008 was 98.4. This number is 26.5 percent higher than the

influenza rate of 2007 and 43.4 percent higher than the

influenza vaccination rate of 2006. Compared to the

National Health Interview Survey rates of influenza

vaccination among health care worker of approximately 35

to 40 percent, the BJC Healthcare's influenza vaccination

rate after implementation of mandatory seasonal influenza vaccination for health care workers is much higher than the national average.

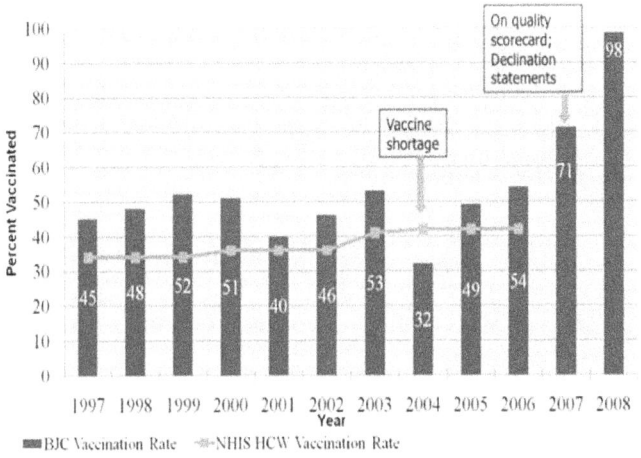

Figure 1. Clinical Infectious Diseases, 2010.

In addition to tracking employee compliance and noncompliance, the occupational health departments tracked employee-reported adverse events. 21 employees cited possible adverse reactions due to the influenza vaccine of varying degrees. The most localized reported adverse reaction was 11 sore arms, while 5 employees reported possible allergic reactions. 4 health care workers reported uncertain reactions, such as fever, muscle pain, upper respiratory symptoms, and a case of a new neurologic condition that could not be positively correlated to the influenza vaccine. In addition, 1 employee reported a possible vagal response and fainting.

Qualitative Results

The BJC Healthcare study reported numerical statistics as well as non-numerical correlations and results of the organization's implementation of mandatory seasonal influenza vaccination of health care workers. For example, the BJC Healthcare study explored factors that contributed to the quantitative success of the 2008 influenza policy implementation, such as communication stressing patient safety and quality of care, management and leadership support of the influenza vaccination policy, and a coordinated campaign across the BJC Healthcare facilities.

In addition, the BJC Healthcare study explored the reasons health care workers requested exemptions.

Although many employees had justified reasons for influenza vaccine exemptions, as demonstrated by occupational health's granting of 411 exemptions, some health care workers did not solely request exemption on the basis of religious or medical causes. BJC Healthcare's employee influenza vaccination policy does not allow declination statements, which in turn does not allow employees to request exemption on the basis of personal opinion. As reported by the BJC Healthcare study, "economic factors at the time of the study may have limited the number of employees willing to lose their jobs."[12]

Moreover, the BJC Healthcare study reported that exemption requests often demonstrated a lack of knowledge or misinformation about the influenza vaccine. To illustrate, several employees requested exemptions due to an immunosuppressed state, which is an indication to receive the influenza vaccine. The request for exemption

---

[12] Hilary M. Babcock and others, eds, "Mandatory Influenza Vaccination of Health Care Workers: Translating Policy to Practice," *Clinical Infectious Diseases*, 50, no. 4 (2010): 459-464, doi: 10.1086/650752.

because of pregnancy, although granted, is not a true

contraindication to the influenza vaccine; rather, pregnant

women are recommended to receive influenza

vaccination.[13]

---

[13] Michele L. Pearson, Carolyn B. Bridges, and Scott A. Harper, "Influenza Vaccination of Health-Care Personnel: Recommendations of the Healthcare Infection Control Practices Advisory Committee (HICPAC) and the Advisory Committee on Immunization Practices (ACIP)," *Morbidity and Mortality Weekly Report*, 55, no. 2 (2006): 1-16, http://www.cdc.gov/mmwr/preview/mmwrhtml/rr5502a1.htm.

CHAPTER 5

DISCUSSION

Introduction

The purpose of this case study was to gain insight into the experiences and issues of implementing mandatory seasonal influenza vaccination policies at health care institutions. This case study sought to explore two primary research questions: whether or not mandatory seasonal influenza vaccination is effective in increasing health care worker coverage of influenza vaccination at health care institutions and what issues or conflicts occur during or after implementation of mandatory seasonal influenza vaccination of health care workers. To explore these two research questions, this case study utilizes inductive data analysis to create patterns, categories, and themes by arranging the data into progressively more abstract divisions of information to form a larger picture of the issue under study. A single-case study based on BJC Healthcare, a large Midwestern health care organization of approximately 26,000 health care workers was selected. Lessons learned through this case study selection are considered relevant and informative about the experiences of implementing mandatory seasonal influenza vaccination for health care workers.

Data collected by BJC Healthcare about the health care organization's influenza vaccination campaigns and the 2008 implementation of mandatory seasonal influenza vaccination policy for health care workers was reviewed in the results sections. In summary, implementation of mandatory seasonal influenza vaccination in 2008 increased health care worker influenza coverage to 98.4 percent. Of the 25,980 health care workers required to receive seasonal influenza vaccination, 25,561 employees received the influenza vaccine, while 411 employees were exempted from influenza vaccination. 99.96 percent of employees, then, were compliant with the mandatory seasonal influenza vaccination policy. The 0.03 percent of employees noncompliant with the influenza vaccination policy were terminated. Thus, the first primary research question of whether or not mandatory seasonal influenza policies increase health care worker influenza coverage was answered positively.

In addition, the BJC Healthcare study explored factors that contributed to the success of the mandatory seasonal influenza vaccination policy for health care workers, including communication stressing patient safety and quality of care, management and leadership support of the influenza vaccination policy, and a coordinated campaign across the BJC Healthcare facilities. Furthermore, the BJC Healthcare study delved into potential reasons health care workers requested exemptions outside of religious or medical reasons. For example, BJC Healthcare's employee influenza vaccination policy does not allow declination statements, which in turn does not allow employees a request for exemption on the basis of personal opinion. As reported by the BJC Healthcare study, "economic factors at the time of the study may have limited the number of employees willing to lose their jobs," and the study also described exemption requests as demonstrating a lack of knowledge or misinformation about the influenza vaccine.[14]

The BJC Healthcare study illustrates the complex nature of implementing mandatory seasonal influenza vaccination policy for health care workers. Although mandatory seasonal influenza vaccination does increase health care worker influenza coverage, implementation of such policy is not straightforward or universally accepted. This section of this case study will examine the nature of the issues of mandatory seasonal influenza vaccination for health care workers at BJC Healthcare and any organization, public or private, that implements mandatory seasonal influenza vaccination policy.

---

[14] Hilary M. Babcock and others, eds, "Mandatory Influenza Vaccination of Health Care Workers: Translating Policy to Practice," *Clinical Infectious Diseases*, 50, no. 4 (2010): 459-464, doi: 10.1086/650752.

Application of Theoretical/Conceptual Framework

This case study utilizes the systems theory as an analytical and conceptual construct to the exploration of mandatory seasonal influenza vaccination. The systems theory, particularly the theory of open systems, appropriately describes the nature of health care and public administration. The purpose of public administration, or the actions carried out by the government to cope with perceived problems through public policies, are influenced by, and concurrently influence, the environment in which they operate.[15] The same simultaneous cycle is also true for health care. Therefore, public administration and similar institutions, such as health care, are open systems according to the systems theory.

Moreover, in any organization, such as public administration and health care, decision-making is made on the basis of goals. In the case of mandatory seasonal

---

[15] Michael C. Lemay, *Public Administration: Clashing Values in the Administration of Public Policy*, 2d ed. (Belmont, CA: Thomson Wadsworth, 2006).

influenza vaccination for health care workers, organizations

center their actions for the purpose of protecting the

public's health and safety. Administrators within these

organizations direct decision processes and make the most

effective choices possible. However, these choices are

complicated by the amount of agreement or disagreement

among decision makers in their attitudes toward the

causation of alternative actions and potential results. In

addition, administrators implementing decisions, such as

mandatory seasonal influenza vaccination, can expect

conflict due to three sources of uncertainty under the

system theory's propositions of Thompson: the labor force,

technology, and the task environment.[16] This construct of

the systems theory can be utilized to explore the second

research question of this study, the issues of mandatory

---

[16] James Thompson, *Organizations in Action: Social Science Bases of Administration Theory* (New York, NY: McGraw-Hill, 1962), quoted in John Miner, *Organizational behavior 2: Essential theories of process and structure* (Armonk, NY: M. E. Sharpe, Inc, 2006). PDF e-book.

seasonal influenza vaccination that occur during or after implementation of policy.

Technology

The first source of uncertainty and conflict in the implementation of mandatory seasonal influenza vaccination policy under the systems theory is technology. Here, the technological aspect of mandatory seasonal influenza vaccination is the influenza vaccine itself. Conflict can arise primarily because of vaccine shortages, which, as the data from the BJC Healthcare study demonstrates, occurred most significantly in 2004.

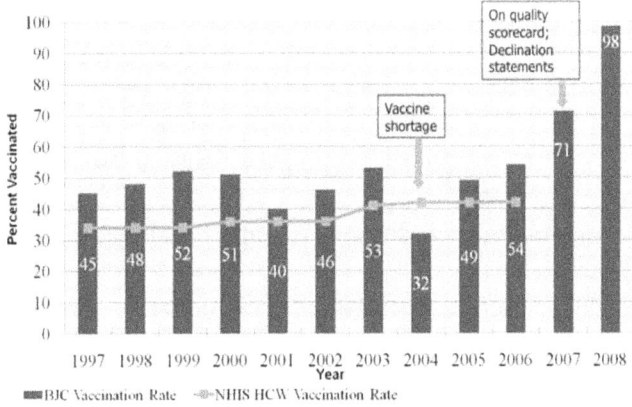

Figure 1. Clinical Infectious Diseases, 2010.

The production and distribution of the influenza vaccine is riddled with potential issues, including a limited number of manufacturers, possible contamination of the vaccine, and the problem of justly distributing the vaccine to the highest risk populations during vaccine shortages. For example, in the 2004-2005 influenza season, the U.S. lost approximately half of its expected vaccine supply when one of the two major manufacturers of the influenza vaccine did not release the vaccine due to potential contamination.[17] Many of the high risk individuals and others in priority groups could not find available vaccinate, including those who were turned away by public and private health care organizations, and never returned when supplies became available.

In a report examining the causes, effects, and actions taken by federal, state, and local health officials during the massive 2004-2005 influenza vaccine shortage,

---

[17, 18] United States Government Accountability Office, "Influenza Vaccine: Shortages in 2004-05 Season Underscore Need for Better Preparation," last modified September 30, 2005, http://www.gao.gov/new.items/d05984.pdf.

the U.S. Government Accountability Office (GAO) stated

that the 2004-2005 influenza season underscored the need

for better preparation. The report cited limited contingency

planning as slowing the government's response; a failure to

expedite actions to boost influenza vaccine's available

supply; and a lack of coordinated communication among

local, state, and federal agencies, which contributed to

delays and confusion and ultimately in a late-season

vaccine surplus.[18] Thus, as evidenced by the 2004-2005

influenza season, technological conflicts can add to

uncertainty in other areas, and human actions taken as a

result of the technological conflict under the systems theory

can cause further issue with voluntary influenza

vaccination and mandatory influenza vaccination.

Labor Force

According to James Thompson, the second source

of uncertainty and conflict under the systems theory is the

---

labor source.[19] The labor source can cause conflict through heterogeneity, or differences in opinions and ideas that affect their performance. For example, the people mandated by a health care organization to receive seasonal influenza vaccination may have opinions or preconceived notions that influence their acceptance of the influenza vaccine. Therefore, in the case of mandatory seasonal influenza vaccination for health care workers, differences of opinions and beliefs among the labor force who are compelled to receive influenza vaccination cause conflict.

In two separate reports, the U.S. Department of Health and Human Services, the Healthcare Infection Control Practices Advisory Committee, and the Advisory Committee on Immunization Practices explored the causes of health care workers' noncompliance with mandatory

---

[19] James Thompson, *Organizations in Action: Social Science Bases of Administration Theory* (New York, NY: McGraw-Hill, 1962), quoted in John Miner, *Organizational behavior 2: Essential theories of process and structure* (Armonk, NY: M. E. Sharpe, Inc, 2006). PDF e-book.

seasonal influenza vaccination.[20, 21] The reports found that many health care workers have personal reasons or fears that prevented their acceptance of the influenza vaccine. These reasons include fear of needles; reliance on homeopathic treatments; lack of physician recommendation; lack of free vaccine; lack of time or convenience; and perceived invulnerability to contracting influenza.

In addition, the reports demonstrated a general lack of knowledge about influenza and the influenza vaccine that stopped health care workers from seeking vaccination, as well as fears about the vaccine. This source of noncompliance include beliefs that influenza is not a serious disease; that the health care worker's own host

---

[20] "HHS Action Plan to Prevent Healthcare-Associated Infections: Influenza Vaccination of Healthcare Personnel," *U.S. Department of Health & Human Services*, last modified May 2010, http://www.hhs.gov/ash/initiatives/hai/tier2_flu.html.

[21] Michele L. Pearson, Carolyn B. Bridges, and Scott A. Harper, "Influenza Vaccination of Health-Care Personnel: Recommendations of the Healthcare Infection Control Practices Advisory Committee (HICPAC) and the Advisory Committee on Immunization Practices (ACIP)," *Morbidity and Mortality Weekly Report*, 55, no. 2 (2006): 1-16, http://www.cdc.gov/mmwr/preview/mmwrhtml/rr5502a1.htm.

defenses will prevent influenza; the belief that the vaccine

is not necessary for people under the age of 65; fear of

contracting influenza-like symptoms from the vaccine; and

fear of vaccine side effects. The reports show that

individual beliefs among health care workers cause a lack

of heterogeneity among the labor force and consequently

conflict to the implementation of mandatory seasonal

influenza vaccination policy.

Task Environment

The last source of uncertainty and conflict under the

systems theory is also the most complex. The task

environment, or, as Thompson defines, the part of the

environment that is not indifferent to an organization,

yields conflict as a result of competing pressures.[22] The

competing pressures in this case study occur in health care

---

[22] James Thompson, *Organizations in Action: Social Science Bases of Administration Theory* (New York, NY: McGraw-Hill, 1962), quoted in John Miner, *Organizational behavior 2: Essential theories of process and structure* (Armonk, NY: M. E. Sharpe, Inc, 2006). PDF e-book.

organizations from supporters and dissenters of mandatory seasonal influenza vaccination for health care workers. These two sides' arguments and conflicts engulf significant and evolving issues that can be divided into two primary categories, ethics and legalities, which will be explored in the following section of this case study.

The decision to implement mandatory seasonal influenza vaccination for health care workers at BJC Healthcare and other health care organizations is founded on ethical arguments. On a larger scale, one can view the mandatory seasonal influenza vaccination regulations as an example of the trade-offs that are central to public policy. As Deborah Stone states, four goals or values direct public policy: security, liberty, efficiency, and equity.[23] In particular, mandatory seasonal influenza vaccination illustrates the changeable scale between liberty and security through the government's responsibility to protect public

---

[23]Deborah Stone, *Policy Paradox: The Art of Political Decision Making*, Revised ed., (New York, NY: W. W. Norton & Company, 2002).

health versus the rights of individuals as protected by law. Ethical arguments for and against mandatory seasonal influenza vaccination can be categorized into two ethical principles: the duty to not harm others and the duty to self.

The duty to not harm others operates under the principle of nonmaleficence and can be viewed as a health care worker's duty to not place his or her patients at undue risk of harm.[24] Applied to mandatory seasonal influenza vaccination, health care workers have a responsibility to their patients to take reasonable steps to stop the transmission of influenza. In addition, mandatory seasonal influenza vaccination would provide health care workers greater immunity and thus increase their capacity to provide care during influenza outbreaks, which would consequently augment beneficence or nonmaleficence.

On the other hand, mandatory seasonal influenza vaccination can be seen as a violation of the duty to self, or

---

[24] Olga Anikeeva, Annette Braunack-Mayer, and Wendy Rogers, "Requiring Influenza Vaccination for Health Care Workers," *Health Policy and Ethics*, 99, no. 1 (2009): 24-29, doi: 10.2105/AJPH.2008.136440.

the right of an individual to carry out his or her own decisions. The ethical principle of autonomy demands a respect for independent decisions and approaches that support the least infringement on individual choice. Mandatory seasonal influenza vaccination is compulsory, which limits the capacity of health care workers to make autonomous decisions about their own health care. Furthermore, in general people have the right to make their own decisions regarding medical care, and compulsion is only used in circumstance in which people are in imminent danger or in which people are incapable of making their own choices.

Neither of these two conditions is met in relation to mandatory seasonal influenza vaccination for health care workers. First, health care workers are competent to make choices about their own medical care. Second, it is challenging to declare that health care workers are a looming danger to the safety of others in the absence of established infection. Compulsion to receive seasonal influenza vaccination, then, infringes on the ethical principle of autonomy and the duty to self.

The ethical arguments presented represent the foundation of the legal issues of mandatory seasonal influenza vaccination. Although no organization has filed a lawsuit against BJC Healthcare in relation to its mandatory seasonal influenza vaccination policy for health care workers, the same cannot be said for other institutions. The first health care institution to implement mandatory seasonal influenza vaccination policy for health care workers was challenged, and this trend has continued for other institutions, as illustrated by the table below.[25] Organizations appealing mandatory seasonal influenza vaccination for health care workers do so on the basis of autonomy and the right to collectively bargain conditions of employment.

---

[25] Wendy Parmet, "Pandemic Vaccines—The Legal Landscape," *The New England Journal of Medicine*, 362, no. 21(2010): 1949-1952, doi:20505176.

Cases Challenging Mandates for Health Care Workers to Receive H1N1 and Seasonal Influenza Vaccines.			
Case Name	Court and Docket Number	Challenged Mandate	Outcome
Brynien v. Daines	N.Y. Sup. Ct. No. 8853–09	New York emergency regulation	Temporary restraining order issued October 16, 2009; state then withdrew regulation and case was dismissed
Patterson v. Daines	N.Y. Sup. Ct. No. 8830–09	New York emergency regulation	Temporary restraining order issued October 16, 2009; state then withdrew regulation and case was dismissed
Savoca v. New York State Dept. of Health	N.Y. Sup. Ct. No. 8855–09	New York emergency regulation	Case dismissed after state withdrew regulation
Field v. Daines	N.Y. Sup. Ct. No. 114033–09	New York emergency regulation	Case dismissed after state withdrew regulation
SEIU Local 121RN v. Healthcare Corp. of America	U.S. Dist. Ct. N.D. Cal. No. 5:09-CV-05065-JF	Hospital's order	Injunction denied on Nov. 17, 2009; parties ordered to submit to arbitration
SEIU Local 1107 v. Southern Hills Medical Center	U.S. Dist. Ct. Nev. No. 2:09-CV-02094-RCJ-PAL	Hospital's order	Temporary restraining order issued halting mandate for seasonal vaccine pending arbitration, Nov. 6, 2009
Washington State Nurses Assoc. v. Multicare Healthcare Systems	U.S. Dist. Ct. W.D. Wash. No. 3:09-CV-05614-RJB	Hospital's order	Temporary restraining order denied; parties agreed to dismiss case

Table 2. The New England Journal of Medicine, 2010.

For example, the Washington State Nurses Association brought a case against Virginia Mason Hospital, the first health care organization to implement mandatory seasonal influenza vaccination for health care workers, as a labor grievance. Arbitrators, including the U.S. Court of Appeals for the 9th Circuit, ruled on behalf of the Washington State Nurses Association. The courts found that personnel of the hospital had the right to collectively bargain over conditions of employment over immunization status because neither federal nor state public health laws required health care worker influenza vaccination as an employment stipulation.[26] After the case was decided, the Washington State Nurses Association negotiated a new influenza control policy with Virginia Mason hospital that did not include dismissal of health care workers that refused seasonal influenza vaccination.

Similarly to *Virginia Mason Hospital vs. Washington State Nurses Association*, health care workers opposed the 2009 New York state regulation that health care workers must receive annual seasonal and H1N1 influenza vaccination. In this situation, health care workers cited that the New York state regulation violated their right to privacy and bodily autonomy; the 14th Amendment due process rights; the right to "freedom of contract" between employee and employer under the 5th and 14th Amendments; and the right to "free exercise" of religion under the 1st Amendment. However, the New York state

---

[26] Alexandra M. Stewart and Sara Rosenbaum, "Law and the Public's Health," *Public Health Reports*, 125, no. 4: 616-618.

regulation was suspended due to influenza vaccine shortage, and the courts summarily dismissed the court cases.

Although opponents of mandatory seasonal influenza vaccination of health care workers have legal support for their arguments, so too do proponents of the policy. For instance, the government has the right to restrict personal liberty to protect the public's health, as demonstrated by *Jacobsen v. Massachusetts*. The U.S. Supreme Court ruled in this case that states have the power to exercise their 10th "Amendment "police powers" to implement vaccination requirements for any group. Furthermore, the courts stated that the health of the public in transmissible disease circumstances outweigh an individual's autonomy and right to refuse health care, which may potentially be applied in the case of influenza vaccination. In addition, the U.S. judicial system has ruled in other court cases that the Contract clause of the Constitution can be nullified by states in the interest of public health and safety, a component of the U.S.

Constitution that health care workers used in New York to

argue against mandatory H1N1 and seasonal influenza

vaccination.

CHAPTER 6

CONCLUSION

This single-case study explored the effectiveness
and issues of implementing mandatory seasonal influenza
vaccination for health care workers at BJC Healthcare, a
large Midwestern health care organization of approximately
26,000 employees. The purpose of this study was to gain
insight into the use, implementation, and issues of
mandatory seasonal influenza vaccination under the
systems theory as a theoretical framework. Using data
collected by BJC Healthcare prior to and after the
implementation of a 2008 mandatory seasonal influenza
vaccination policy for health care workers, this case study
found that mandatory seasonal influenza vaccination for
health care workers does increase influenza vaccine
coverage at health care organizations. However, as the
qualitative results of this study demonstrate, conflict arises

as a result of the mandatory seasonal influenza vaccination policy.

By applying the systems theory to the results of the BJC study, this case study categorized the issues of mandatory seasonal influenza vaccination into three categories of uncertainty and conflict: technology, the labor force, and the task environment. Each division of conflict exhibited several areas of uncertainty that complicate the implementation of mandatory seasonal influenza vaccination of health care workers, and according to the systems theory, resolution of conflict must occur to meet optimal organization function and effectiveness.[27] Therefore, in the case of mandatory seasonal influenza vaccination of health care workers, health care institutions need to address the three sources of conflict.

---

[27] James Thompson, *Organizations in Action: Social Science Bases of Administration Theory* (New York, NY: McGraw-Hill, 1962), quoted in John Miner, *Organizational behavior 2: Essential theories of process and structure* (Armonk, NY: M. E. Sharpe, Inc, 2006). PDF e-book.

The first source of uncertainty or conflict, technology, primarily creates conflict through the influenza vaccine, specifically influenza vaccine shortages. As the GAO report summarizes, influenza vaccine shortages cause many high risk and priority individuals to not receive influenza vaccination, and actions taken by federal, local, and state health officials exacerbated the situation in the 2004-2005 influenza season.[28] Thus, in order to resolve conflict due to technology under the systems theory in the case of mandatory seasonal influenza vaccination, health care institutions would need to find ways to increase influenza vaccine supply and create effective contingency and communication plans that would facilitate vaccine supply availability to high risk and priority populations.

Under the systems theory, the second source of conflict is the labor force. In the case of mandatory seasonal influenza vaccination of health care workers, the

[28] United States Government Accountability Office, "Influenza Vaccine: Shortages in 2004-05 Season Underscore Need for Better Preparation," last modified September 30, 2005, http://www.gao.gov/new.items/d05984.pdf.

labor source can produce conflict through a lack of homogeneity regarding health care workers' acceptance, personal fears and opinions, and preconceived notions about influenza and the influenza vaccine.[29,30] Therefore, health care organizations must seek to facilitate heterogeneity in the labor source to resolve conflict. For example, health care organizations could hold educational meetings or campaigns that emphasize the benefits of health care worker influenza vaccination for staff and patients and dispel myths about influenza and the influenza vaccine.

Lastly, health care organizations need to address the final source of conflict under the systems theory, the task environment. The task environment fosters conflict

---

[29] "HHS Action Plan to Prevent Healthcare-Associated Infections: Influenza Vaccination of Healthcare Personnel," *U.S. Department of Health & Human Services*, last modified May 2010, http://www.hhs.gov/ash/initiatives/hai/tier2_flu.html.
[30] Michele L. Pearson, Carolyn B. Bridges, and Scott A. Harper, "Influenza Vaccination of Health-Care Personnel: Recommendations of the Healthcare Infection Control Practices Advisory Committee (HICPAC) and the Advisory Committee on Immunization Practices (ACIP)," *Morbidity and Mortality Weekly Report*, 55, no. 2 (2006): 1-16, http://www.cdc.gov/mmwr/preview/mmwrhtml/rr5502a1.htm.

through ethical and legal arguments for and against

mandatory seasonal influenza vaccination of health care

workers. Although both supporters and dissenters of

mandatory seasonal influenza vaccination policies of health

care workers have ethical and legal support for their

arguments, judicial ruling to date has ruled in favor of

individual autonomy.[31] However, as *Jacobsen v.*

Massachusetts demonstrates, future rulings could shift in

favor of public health over individual rights, or security

over liberty. Until a conclusive judicial decision is

reached, however, the conflict caused by the task

environment will not be resolved.

In conclusion, mandatory seasonal influenza

vaccination for health care workers is effective in

increasing health care worker influenza coverage.

Increased influenza vaccination translates into decreased

incidence of nosocomial influenza infection and better

patient outcomes. However, as this case study shows, the

---

[31] Alexandra M. Stewart and Sara Rosenbaum, "Law and the Public's Health," *Public Health Reports*, 125, no. 4: 616-618.

promotion of public health through mandatory seasonal influenza vaccination of health care workers infringes on individual rights and autonomy, and the implementation of mandatory seasonal influenza vaccination policy of health care workers creates other avenues of conflict. Under the systems theory, these issues can be categorized into three sources of conflict: technology, the labor force, and the task environment. In order to resolve conflict, then, organizations must address these three sources of conflict and uncertainty to promote optimal organizational effectiveness and function. Therefore, health care institutions, in collaboration with public and judicial support, need to explore ways in which to settle arguments over the issues of mandatory seasonal influenza vaccination of health care workers to support widespread acceptance and successful implementation of mandatory seasonal influenza vaccination of health care workers.

BIBLIOGRAPHY

Anikeeva, Olga, Braunack-Mayer, Annette, and Wendy Rogers. "Requiring Influenza Vaccination for Health Care Workers." *Health Policy and Ethics*, 99, no. 1 (2009): 24-29. doi: doi: 10.2105/AJPH.2008.136440.

Babcock, Hilary M., Gemeinhart, Nancy, Jones, Marilyn, Dunagan, Claiborne, and Keith F. Woeltje. "Mandatory Influenza Vaccination of Health Care Workers: Translating Policy into Practice." *Clinical Infectious Diseases*, 50, no. 4 (2010): 459-464. doi: 10.1086/650752.

Creswell, John W. *Research Design: Qualitative, Quantitative, and Mixed Methods Approaches*, 3d ed. Los Angeles, CA: SAGE Publications, Inc., 2009.

"HHS Action Plan to Prevent Healthcare-Associated Infections: Influenza Vaccination of Healthcare Personnel." *U.S. Department of Health & Human Services*. Last modified May 2010. http://www. Hhs.gov/ash/initiatives/hai/tier2_flu.html.

Katz, Daniel, and Robert L. Kahn. "Organizations and the Systems Concept." In *Classics of Public Administration*, 6h ed., ed Jay M. Shafritz and Albert Hyde. Boston, MA: Thomson Wadsworth, 2007.

LeMay, Michael C. *Public Administration: Clashing Values in the Administration of Public Policy*, 2d ed. Belmont, CA: Thomson Wadsworth, 2006.

Parmet, Wendy. "Pandemic Vaccines—The Legal Landscape." *The New England Journal of Medicine*, 362, no. 21 (2010): 1949-1952. doi: 20505176.

Pearson, Michele L., Bridges, Carolyn B., and Scott A. Harper. "Influenza Vaccination of Health-Care Personnel: Recommendations of the Healthcare Infection Control Practices Advisory Committee (HICPAC) and the Advisory Committee on Immunization Practices (ACIP)." *Morbidity and Mortality Weekly*, 55, no. 2 (2006): 1-16. doi: 2010-623-026/41266.

"Seasonal Influenza (Flu)." *Centers for Disease Control and Prevention*. Last modified September 15, 2010. http://www.cdc.gov/flu.

Stewart, Alexandra M., and Sara Rosenbaum. "Law and the Public's Health," *Public Health Report*, 125, no. 4: 616-618.

Stone, Deborah. *Policy Paradox: The Art of Political Decision Making*, revised ed. New York, NY: W. W. Norton & Company, 2002.

Talbot, Thomas R., and William Schaffner. "On Being the First: Virginia Mason Medical Center and Mandatory Influenza vaccination of Healthcare workers." *Infection Control Hospital Epidemiology*, 31, no. 9 (2010): 889-892. doi: 10.10.1086/656211.

Thompson, James. *Organizations in Action: Social Sciences Bases of Administration Theory*. New York, NY: McGraw-Hill, 1962. Quoted in John Miner, *Organizational behavior 2: Essential theories of process and structure*. Armonk, NY: M. E. Sharpe, Inc., 2006. PDF e-book.

U.S. Government Accountability Office. "Influenza
　　Vaccine: Shortages in 2004-2005 Season
　　Underscore Need for Better Preparation." Last
　　modified September 30, 2005.
　　http://www.gao.gov/new.items/d05984.pdf.

www.ingramcontent.com/pod-product-compliance
Lightning Source LLC
Chambersburg PA
CBHW051241170526
45165CB00004B/1518